Disclaimer

Before beginning any exercise or nutrition programme, please
consult with your doctor to make sure you are in good health.
This manual is not meant to replace proper medical advice by a
qualified health practitioner. No liability is assumed by ABC fit or
Aaron Breckell for any of the information contained in this
document.

Published by ABC fit

All rights reserved. No part of this document may be reproduced,
distributed, or transmitted in any form or by any means, including
photocopying, recording, or other electronic or mechanical
methods, without the prior written permission of the publisher.

www.abcfit.co.uk

Contents

Your Time Is Now 01
Before You Begin 03
Tracking Progress 04
Sharpen Up! Class In Session... 05
A = EXERCISE 06
Exercise Basics For Building Muscle 07
A Word On Warming-Up 08
Understanding The Programme Cards 09
Phase One 10
Workouts A/B 11
Phase Two 12
Workouts C/D 13
Workouts E/F 14
Exercise Descriptions 15
Home Adaptations 23
B = NUTRITION 24
The Seven Principles Of Nutrition 25
Supplements 31
A Day In The Life 32
The 80/20 Rule 33
C = RECOVERY 34
Sleep Fundamentals 35
Active Recovery 36
The Active Recovery Session 37
FAQs 39
Basic Anatomy 41
Enjoyed The Programme? 42
Maximise Your Results 43
About ABC fit 44

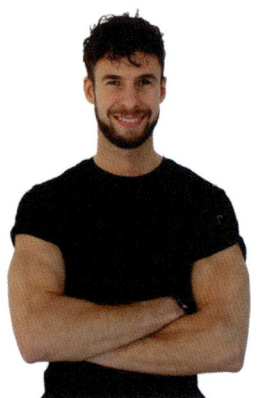

"From the bottom of my heart - Thank you. Thank you for investing into ABC fit to help with your health and fitness goals. I'm excited for you to get stuck in to this manual and more importantly being empowered to move forward and start seeing results!"

Aaron Breckell

Cover image: Pexels.com

www.abcfit.co.uk

Your Time Is Now!

I had just one aim with this training guide.

To create the source of knowledge I so badly needed when I was in my teens.

You see it took me years to understand how to build muscle and eat for my goals. This was made much worse by the fact I was learning my info from bodybuilding magazines which were aimed at either A) Very experienced lifters or B) Lifters on steriods or C) Both! Neither of which applied to me.

Finding useful content for "teens looking to build muscle" was tough.

With this guide, I wanted to create the ultimate resource for any teen looking to build some muscle and live a healthier, happier more confident life. Consider this guide your ticket to fast tracking the years of trail and error I had to endure as a teen.

The good news is as a teen your body is primed to build muscle rapidly! Your hormones such as testosterone (the king of muscle building hormones!) are surging, your energy levels are buzzing and your appetite is up. You just need to create a stimulus through training and eat for your goals, both of which you're going to learn how to do over the pages to come. Your time is now!

My ethos with all things fitness has always been simplicity and sustainability. To be able to take an otherwise complicated topic such as building muscle and break it down into the facts you need to know, and combining that with measures that ensure you can sustain the behaviours forever, is important to me.

This is why The 8 Week Teen Muscle Project is different from other training programmes you may have come across before. The behaviours introduced over the 8 weeks are simple, effective and most importantly, sustainable. As far as I'm concerned, this is the only workout or nutrition plan you'll need to help you put on high quality muscle mass gains in your teenage years.

So I think its time for me to introduce The 8 Week Teen Muscle Project. Across the following pages the manual is divided into three main sections:

A - Exercise

B - Nutrition

C - Recovery

www.abcfit.co.uk

Each section in the guide will give you a specific set of instructions. Follow them closely and you'll:

- Learn how to build mass and strengthen and define your muscles through the correct training protocols.

- Provide your body with the nutrients you need to build lean tissue and sustain energy levels!

- Uncover the various techniques that will speed up the recovery process and keep your tissues and joints healthy.

All of the protocols outlined throughout this guide have been tried and tested out in the field countless times by myself and my extensive range of clientele. Each section of the guide is designed to work in harmony with the other, so ensure you're combining step A, B and C together to the best of your ability. Understand that you are the only person who can hold you back. So stop the excuses, work hard and you'll reap the rewards of success. It's time to make a big decision - are you ready to build some muscle? OK then let's do this! Enjoy the next 8 weeks, it's going to be an incredible journey.

Your coach,

Aaron Breckell

"The only impossible journey is the one you never begin."
Anthony Robbins

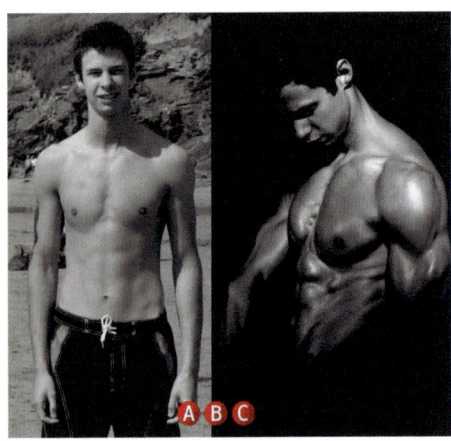

My "teen muscle building" transformation. 18 years old versus 20 years old...

www.abcfit.co.uk

Before You Begin

Before you begin, it's important to set some goals for the next 8 weeks. Without a goal you can focus on and work towards, your progress will suffer. So grab a pen and paper and let's set some goals.

Goal Setting

SMART goal
A SMART goal is Specific, Measurable, Achievable, Realistic and Time-bound. Since this is a 8 week plan, let's set an 8 week goal. Healthy muscle gain is around 1-2lb per month. As you're new to training you may see gains faster than this. So work out how much you want to gain and jot it down.

Benefits
Imagine yourself 8 weeks from now. You've achieved your goal, how is this going to benefit you? How are you going to look and feel?

Challenges
What challenges are you going to face over the next 8 weeks?

Solutions
What are your challenges? Let's have a think about potential solutions you could implement this week that will help eradicate them. Here's some of the most common challenges I hear with a corresponding solution.

Lack of time - better diary planning.
Wrong food choices - read section B and educate yourself on better food choices.
Partying - limit partying to 1-2 times per month.

www.abcfit.co.uk

Tracking Progress

If your goal is SMART, it should be measurable. I would strongly urge you to pick two or more methods below to track your progress. Perform a re-test every 2-4 weeks to ensure the changes you're seeing are for the better. If they're not, that's fine. You just need to work out why and what you can do to change that.

Body Photos
Wear as little clothing as possible and take from front, side and back. When you come to take a second batch of progress photos, make sure you're in the same room with the same lighting.

Weight
Use an accurate set of scales in pounds or kilograms. When you come to do a progress check use the same scales on the same type of flooring. Bioelectrical Impedance Analysis (BIA) scales, such as those made by Tanita are also great for estimating your body composition.

Body Fat Calliper Test
This is a great way of determining your body fat percentage. Since the aims of this plan are to help you build muscle, this number should not be increasing too much. Seek a trained fitness professional to perform the test.

Circumference Measurements
Pick body parts including calves, thighs, waist, chest, arms and neck and take a circumference measurement in centimetres or inches. This is a great way to see where you're making gains.

Record Your Workouts
It doesn't matter whether you use your mobile, a tablet or even just good old fashioned pen and paper, you need to be recording your workouts. To see optimal results from this training plan you need to be applying what's known as progressive overload. This is a gradual increase in training stress placed on the body. In other words, each consecutive workout you should be striving to lift a little more, decrease the rest periods or perform more reps. This is where recording your workouts comes in handy because you can see exactly what you did last time. Be sure to record the following:

- Date and time of workout
- Exercise/sets/reps completed
- Weights used
- Time taken to complete the session

www.abcfit.co.uk

Sharpen up! Class In Session...

One of the biggest questions I probably get from the average teenager looking to start working out is "How do I fit it all in around my studies?". I'm sure many of you reading this are at school or college, so this will be really important for you.

Now I don't want to start sounding like your parents. I'm sure you're sick of hearing how important your schooling and education is blah blah blah. But seriously it is, you only get one shot at it so it should remain a top priority for you.

With that said, working out and having goals to build muscle and gain strength can actually help you. Think about it - training and eating a good diet will help de-stress you and build confidence which will cross over into how you act and react around school or college.

Getting your workouts in around the school or college day is actually easier than you might think, you just need to use initiative and plan ahead. As you'll come to see, the workouts are periodised into two phases. Phase one is made up of three sessions per week, whereas phase two increases up to four per week. Each session will take around 45-60 minutes to complete. So neither is unrealistic in the grand scheme of things. One tip I'd encourage you to do is to look at your week every Monday and plan in when you want to actually get your workouts in. Remember you can train in the morning before school starts. You could do a lunch time session if there's time. Or you could do after school in the evening. There's no real "right way" just get your session in when you can/when feels best.

And what about extra curricular activities I hear you say? Things like sports, such as football or tennis can compliment your weights sessions nicely. I'd limit it to no more than 2-3 sessions per week. Too much could distract you (mentally and physically!), meaning you won't get the most out of this plan. Even creative extra curricular activities such as art or music could help you unwind and destress from the ups and downs of full-time education.

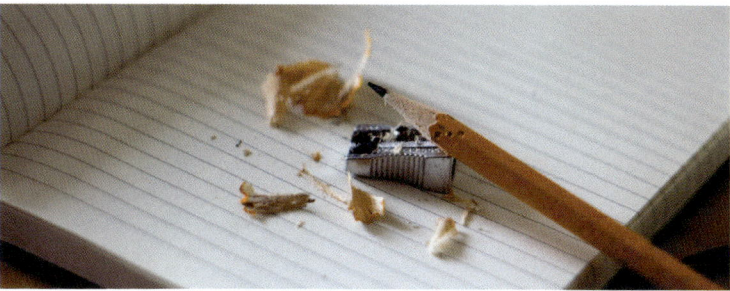

www.abcfit.co.uk

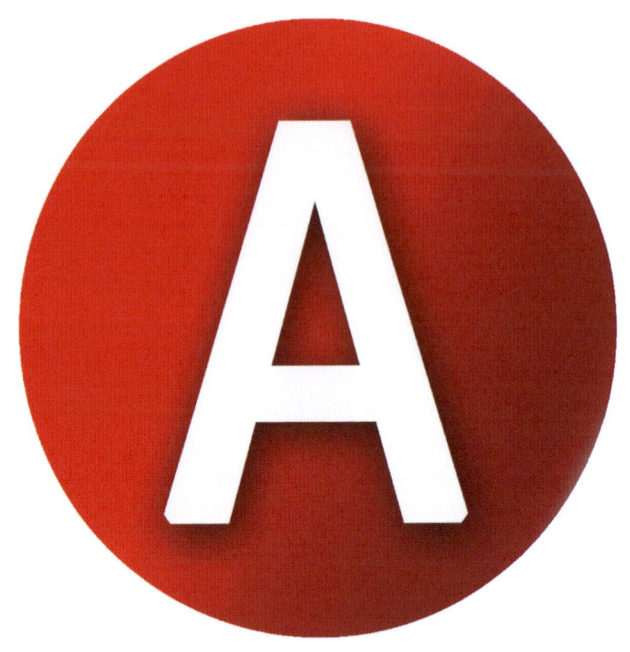

A = EXERCISE

Activity requiring physical effort, carried out to sustain or improve health and fitness

Exercise Basics For Building Muscle

Let's get the boring science out of the way. If you're looking for increased muscle size, you need to go into the gym with a specific purpose. If every workout has a purpose then you will adapt and grow. Time and time again, research has confirmed heavy resistance training is the most effective method for building tissue. The reason being, heavy weight stimulates the type II muscle fibres; these are the ones with most potential for growth.

So we understand heavy resistance training is a good place to start for increasing muscle size, but if we start to dig deeper there's three major pathways that actually induce this hypertrophy. According to Brad Schoenfeld in The Journal of Strength and Conditioning Research, mechanical tension, muscle damage and metabolic stress are the factors that will induce the results you desire.

Mechanical tension is a result of heavy resistance training. It is created by muscle stretch, strict form and heavy weights. Increased weight isn't the be-all and end-all of maximising tension though. The tempo or speed at which you perform an exercise canmake a huge difference. A five-second eccentric (negative portion of the rep) will certainly jack up the tension!

Increased mechanical tension is very efficient at doing muscle damage. Around two days after a workout your DOMS (Delayed Onset Muscle Soreness) will likely reach its peak. This soreness is somewhat indicative of the amount of damage you did. Damage is created by doing something unfamiliar to the body. This could be more weight, more reps, reduced rest periods or an alternative tempo etc. Otherwise known as progressive overload. The human body desires a state of homeostasis. When this pattern of balance is interrupted, adaptations will take place.

Metabolic stress results from several factors including:

- The hypoxia or lack of oxygen supply to the muscles during a set.
- The trapping of blood in the muscle that creates the swelling look and the feeling that many bodybuilders chase, known as "the pump".
- The by-products of anaerobic metabolism, such as lactate build-up and the increased hormonal surge that goes with it.

There we have it, three factors that all go hand-in-hand for maximum gains. If you take home one point from this section - don't judge the effectiveness of a workout on how much weight you just moved, but rather how much mechanical tension, muscle damage and metabolic stress you created. Followed correctly the workouts over the next 8 weeks will effectively stimulate your muscles through these pathways.

www.abcfit.co.uk

A Word On Warming-Up

Just like you can't hop in a super car and expect it to be able to perform at its best without first warming the engine, your body also needs to be warm for it to perform optimally. Many people arrive at the gym and just go straight into their first set, which is a big mistake. A good warm-up has many important purposes:

- Promotes blood flow to the muscles.
- Injury prevention.
- Lubricates the joints and tissues for better range of motion.
- Switches on the central nervous system for better muscle recruitment and a more effective workout.

The warm-up I recommend for The 8 Week Teen Muscle Project workouts will take no more than ten minutes. It's split into two parts:

Part One
General CV - Choose from treadmill, cross trainer, rower or bike and perform at a steady pace for five minutes. Instead of just climbing on and aimlessly pedaling, get your mind in the zone. Think about what you want to achieve during the workout. Going in with a laser-guided focus like this will almost always result in a better quality session.

Part Two
Dynamic movements - The three dynamic movement patterns shown below are there to mobilise the shoulders, spine, hips and knees. All common areas that are at a high risk of injury during physical activity. Perform each one at a slow and steady pace and once completed you'll be ready to begin your workout.

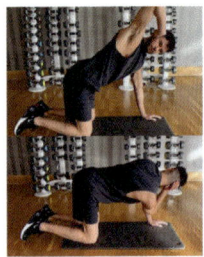

Quadruped T-spine rotations
12 per side

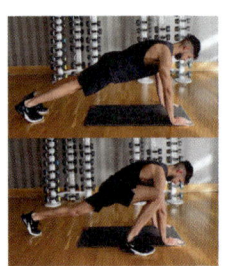

Mountain climbers
20 reps

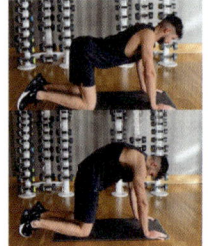

Cat camels
10 reps

www.abcfit.co.uk

Understanding The Programme Cards

The programme card is an extremely effective and simple way to prescribe exercise. This page guides you through the basics of using and reading the programme cards.

The workout name is displayed at the top.

Exercises are displayed down the left side.

Tempo - determines the speed at which you should perform an exercise. It is displayed using four digits.
- 1st digit: seconds on the eccentric.
- 2nd digit: seconds on the pause at the bottom.
- 3rd digit: seconds on the concentric.
- 4th digit: seconds on the pause at the top.

Workout A:

EXERCISE	SETS	REPS	TEMPO	REST	NOTES
1: barbell squat	4	8	4010	90 sec	1: warm up with 2-3 lighter sets
2A: walking dumbell lunges	3	20	2010	5 sec	
2B: kb swing	3	40 sec	1010	60 sec	
3A: crunch	2	12	2010	5 sec	3A: add weight if needed
3B: hanging leg raise	2	12	2010	5 sec	
3C: plank	2	60 sec	NA	60 sec	

Sets - how many blocks of reps you should perform.

Rest - how long to rest between sets.

Reps - how many times you perform the movement in a given set.

Numbers and letters indicate the order you should perform exercises. In this example, a walking lunge is performed followed by a leg extension with five seconds rest between exercises. After both exercises have been performed, you would then rest for 60 seconds and repeat for sets.

Notes - provide specific information you may need to know for various exercises.

www.abcfit.co.uk

Phase One (Weeks 1-4)

Phase Focus: Building A Foundation

Welcome to phase one of the plan. Here we are going to be alternating between two full-body resistance sessions - Workout A and Workout B. The two sessions are based on full body sessions and our main aim over the next four weeks is to build some foundational strength and muscle.

I know - I bet you're thinking what about the "bro split"? All my mates train chest on monday, back on tuesday etc. Well let me tell you, the "bro split" was one of my biggest training mistakes I made when first starting out. It's not wrong there's just better ways to go about it. Full body sessions are just one way. There's two very important reasons why that you need to know about. The first reason is that by using a full body split you increase the frequency a particular muscle is trained. In this case each muscle will be stimulated three times per week. And remember the more you can stimulate a muscle to grow, the more growth you will experience.

Reason number two is that you have the ability to maximise total muscle recruitment during a full body workout and this means more muscle built and a better hormonal environment for maximum gains.

There's no bells or whistles to these workouts. They're just bread and butter workouts for building a strong foundation.

Be smart when selecting a loads - Don't lift with your ego! Look to progress these sessions over the coming four weeks by striving to lift more load for the desired number of reps and sets.

Weekly Training Schedule

Week 1,3:
- Mon - Workout A
- Tue - Rest day
- Wed - Workout B
- Thur - Rest day
- Fri - Workout A
- Sat & Sun - Rest day

Week 2,4:
- Mon - Workout B
- Tue - Rest day
- Wed - Workout A
- Thur - Rest day
- Fri - Workout B
- Sat & Sun - Rest day

www.abcfit.co.uk

Workout A: Full Body

EXERCISE	SETS	REPS	TEMPO	REST	NOTES
1: BB Squat	4	8-10	3010	60 sec	Strive for the higher number of each given rep bracket (8-10 reps, go for 10 reps). If you complete all sets with the higher figure, increase the weight next time.
2: Back Extension Bench	4	8-10	2020	60 sec	
3: Press up	4	8-10	3010	60 sec	
4: One Arm DB Row	4	8-10	3010	60 sec	
5: Plank	4	30-60s	NA	30 sec	

Workout B: Full Body

EXERCISE	SETS	REPS	TEMPO	REST	NOTES
1: BB Deadlift	5	4-6	2010	90 sec	Strive for the higher number of each given rep bracket (8-10 reps, go for 10 reps). If you complete all sets with the higher figure, increase the weight next time.
2; Leg Press	4	8-10	3010	60 sec	
3: Seated Pulldown	4	8-10	3010	60 sec	
4: Seated DB press	4	8-10	3010	60 sec	
5: BB curl	3	12-15	2010	60 sec	

Please Note: Terms throughout the plan have been shortened to save space.

BB = Barbell
DB = Dumbbell
AMAP = As many as possible

www.abcfit.co.uk

Phase Two (Weeks 5-8)

Phase Focus: Shifting Up A Gear

During this second phase of training (Weeks 5-8), you'll notice the workouts now adopt a lower/upper style split. This allows you to direct more volume into each muscle group and will really mix up your training. You'll probably be feeling a little sore and stiff the after the first couple of sessions, so it's paramount you nail your nutrition and sleep to recover as fast as possible. With this, expect your gains to grow a new lease of life!

Again we focus on straight sets, keeping things nice and simple. But remember simple doesn't mean in-effective. You'll also notice a few new exercises creeping in here and there. So be sure to double check your form agaisnt the "exercise descriptions" section later in the guide.

Once again you should be looking to progressively overload your body with these workouts. We can do this by lifting more load for the desired number of reps, but remember don't do this at the expense of solid, strict form. Also don't forget the tempos listed with each exercise. Remember this refers to the speed at which we perform a given exercise.

Before you get cracking with the next phase of workouts, I just wanted to remind you that I am always here for questions and support during your journey. You can email me at info@abcfit.co.uk or DM me direct via any of my social media channels (which I hope you are following by now!).

Weekly Training Schedule

Weeks 5,6,7,8:
Mon - Workout C (lower)
Tue - Workout D (upper)
Wed - Rest Day
Thur - Workout E (lower)
Fri - Workout F (upper)
Sat & Sun - Rest day

www.abcfit.co.uk

Workout C: Lower Body

EXERCISE	SETS	REPS	TEMPO	REST	NOTES
1: BB Squat	4	12-15	3010	60 sec	Strive for the higher number of each given rep bracket (12-15 reps, go for 15 reps). If you complete all sets with the higher figure, increase the weight next time.
2: Back Extension Bench	4	12-15	3010	60 sec	
3: Leg Extension	4	12-15	2010	60 sec	
4: DB Lunges	3	20-30	2010	60 sec	
5: Seated Twist	3	20-30	2010	60 sec	

Workout D: Upper Body

EXERCISE	SETS	REPS	TEMPO	REST	NOTES
1: Flat BB Press	4	12-15	3010	60 sec	Strive for the higher number of each given rep bracket (12-15 reps, go for 15 reps). If you complete all sets with the higher figure, increase the weight next time.
2: Seated Pulldown	4	12-15	3010	60 sec	
3: Cable Fly	4	12-15	3010	60 sec	
4: BB curl	3	12-15	3010	60 sec	
5: Rope Pressdown	3	12-15	3010	60 sec	

Please Note: Terms throughout the plan have been shortened to save space.

BB = Barbell
DB = Dumbbell
AMAP = As many as possible

www.abcfit.co.uk

Workout E: Lower Body

EXERCISE	SETS	REPS	TEMPO	REST	NOTES
1: DB Romanian Deadlift	4	12-15	3010	60 sec	Strive for the higher number of each given rep bracket (12-15 reps, go for 15 reps). If you complete all sets with the higher figure, increase the weight next time.
2: Leg press	4	12-15	3010	60 sec	
3: Seated Leg curl	4	12-15	3010	60 sec	
4: DB Lunges	3	20-30	2010	60 sec	
5: Crunch	3	15-20	2020	60 sec	

Workout F: Upper Body

EXERCISE	SETS	REPS	TEMPO	REST	NOTES
1: One Arm DB Row	4	12-15	3010	60 sec	Strive for the higher number of each given rep bracket (12-15 reps, go for 15 reps). If you complete all sets with the higher figure, increase the weight next time.
2: Seated DB Press	4	12-15	3010	60 sec	
3: DB Rear Delt Fly	4	12-15	2010	60 sec	
4: DB Hammer Curl	3	12-15	2020	60 sec	
5: Close Grip Push-up	3	AMAP	2010	60 sec	

Please Note: Terms throughout the plan have been shortened to save space.

BB = Barbell
DB = Dumbbell
AMAP = As many as possible

www.abcfit.co.uk

Exercise Descriptions

Here you will find a description of the exercises used throughout the 8 week programme. Coaching cues are given for some exercises, these are important points you need to understand if you want to get the most out of the exercise.

Lower Body

Barbell Back Squat
Target Areas: Quads, Glutes, Hamstrings

With a bar across the top of your shoulders and a firm grip on the bar, keep your back flat and push your hamstrings and glutes back. As you sit down into the squat keep your chest and head up. When you reach end-range, drive through your heels and stand back up.

Coaching Cue - Drive your knees out.

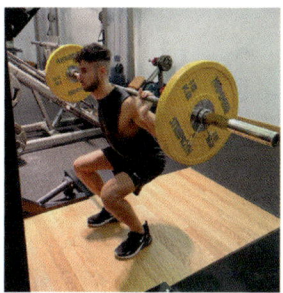

Dumbbell Romanian Deadlift
Target Areas: Hamstrings, Glutes

Hold a pair of dumbbells at arms length around the front of your body. With knees slighty soft hinge at the hip, tipping forward. Be sure to keep your spine tall and chest up during the movement.

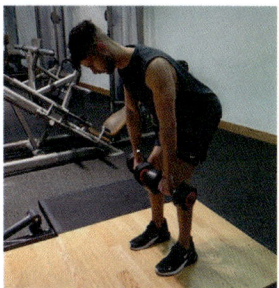

Dumbbell Lunge
Target Areas: Quads, Hamstrings, Glutes

Holding a pair of dumbbells at your sides stand up tall and take a step forward into the lunge. The front knee should be bent at 90 degrees in the bottom position. Be sure not to let your back knee smash into the ground in the bottom position.

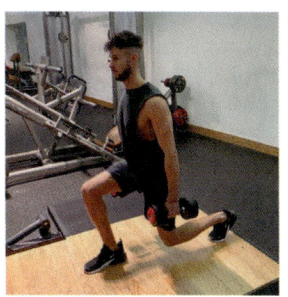

www.abcfit.co.uk

Leg Press
Target Areas: Quads, Hamstrings, Glutes

Using a leg press machine, lower the weight under control until end range. Your pelvis shouldn't be coming off the seat in this position. If it is, you're going too low. Press back up to the top and be sure to keep the knees slightly soft. This helps to protect the knee joint.

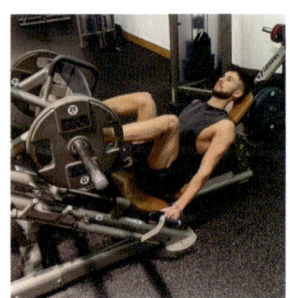

Barbell Deadlift
Target Areas: Hamstrings, Glutes, Back

This is a great exercise for hitting everything along the posterior chain. Holding a barbell at arms length, hinge at the hip until you feel a stretch in the hamstrings. Reverse this motion and stand back up to finish the rep. Ensure you keep your back flat and core engaged with this one.

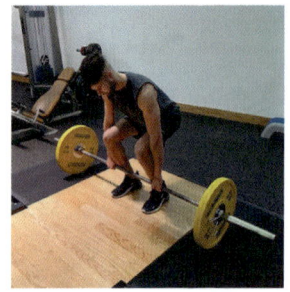

Back Extension Bench
Target Areas: Glutes, Hamstrings

Using a 45 degree back extension bench, keep your back flat and hinge at the hip until you can feel a stretch in your hamstrings. Once you reach end-range, return back up to the start to finish the rep. Please note the body is straight at the starting position, not hyperextended.

Coaching Cue - To get the most out of this exercise, aim for a stretch of the hams in the bottom position and a squeeze of the glutes at the top.

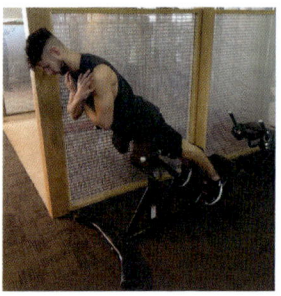

Seated Leg Curl
Target Areas: Hamstrings

Get yourself set up on seated leg curl machine. Flex your knee to at least 90 degrees and squeeze your hamstrings before lowering the weight back to the starting position. This is a great exercise to isolate the hamstrings.

Coaching Cue - Be careful not to point your toes when performing this exercise, or else you'll just feel it on your calves as you contract them.

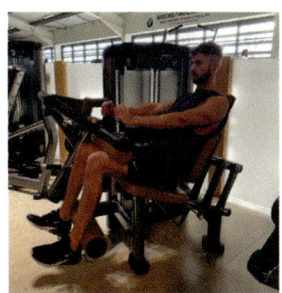

Leg Extension
Target Areas: Quads

Get yourself set up on leg extension machine. Extend your knee to the top and squeeze your quads before lowering the weight back to the starting position. This is a great exercise to isolate the quads. Feel the burn!

Coaching Cue - Keep your feet pointing straight with this one.

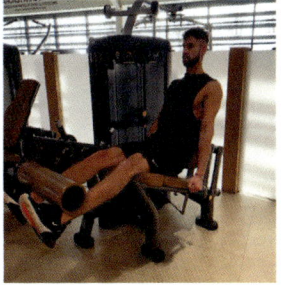

Upper Body

Seated Dumbbell Press
Target Areas: Delts, Triceps

Start by holding a pair of dumbbells slightly wider than shoulder width grip at chest height. Press them directly above your head. Carefully lower to the starting position. Keep your core squeezed throughout this one to keep your spine safe and posture correct.

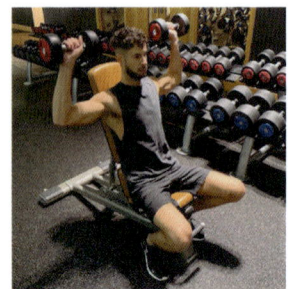

Flat Barbell Press
Target Areas: Pecs, Delts, Triceps

Lie on a flat bench press and grab the bar slightly wider than shoulder width apart. Lower the bar under control to the the mid chest before pressing it back up to the starting position. Keep your elbows slightly off lock to keep constant tension on the muscles.

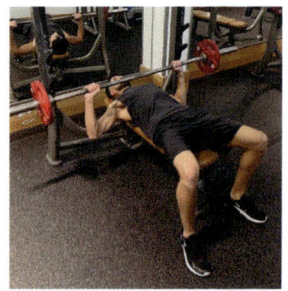

Cable Flye
Target Areas: Pecs

Set a cable stack to around head height. Grab the handles and take a step into it. With the eblows slightly soft, but fixed, open the chest up until you feel a slight stretch across the chest muscles. Remember to just move from the shoulder joint. The elbow shouldn't flex. Return back to the start of the movement.

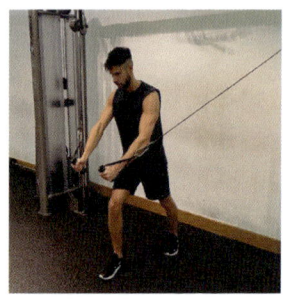

Dumbbell Rear Delt Raise
Target Areas: Rear Delts

Grab two lighter dumbbells and hinge at the hip. Whilst keeping your back flat. perform almost like the reverse of a flye movement.

Coaching Cue - Keep the spine flat and don't jolt to cheat. Also don't allow the dumbbells to touch. This keeps tension on the working muscles.

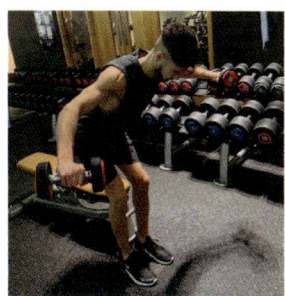

Seated Pulldown
Target Areas: Lats, Biceps

Take a seat on a lat pulldown machine and grab the handles with a slightly wider than shoulder width grip. Pull the bar down to the top of your chest, squeezing your shoulder blades together, before returning to the start.

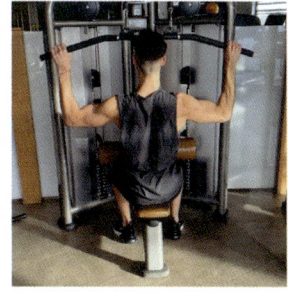

One Arm Dumbbell Row
Target Areas: Lats, Rhomboids, Biceps

Place one knee and one arm on a bench. Whilst keeping your spine flat row (pull) the dumbbell up towards the side of the chest. Squeeze the shoulder blade at the top, before lowering the weight back to the start.

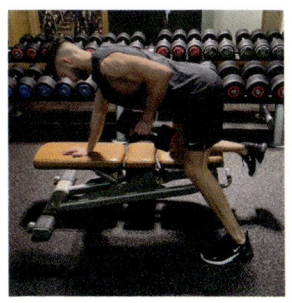

www.abcfit.co.uk

Press Up
Target Areas: Pecs, Delts, Triceps

Place hands slightly wider than shoulder width apart. lower your self to the ground and then push back up the start. Keep the glutes and core braced throughout.

Coaching Cue - Can also be performed from the knees for an easier option.

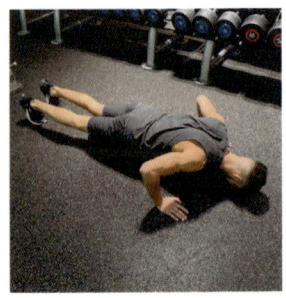

Close Grip Push Up
Target Areas: Delts, Triceps

Performed as above, but with hands around 6 inches apart.

Coaching Cue - Keep the core engaged and elbows tucked in to the sides.

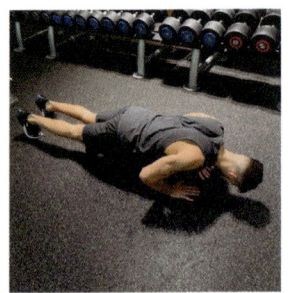

Barbell Curl
Target Areas: Biceps

Stand tall and hold a bar, palms facing forward. Keeping the elbows fixed into your sides, curl the bar up to your chest. Squeeze the biceps to ensure recruitment. Remember to keep it controlled on the way back down.

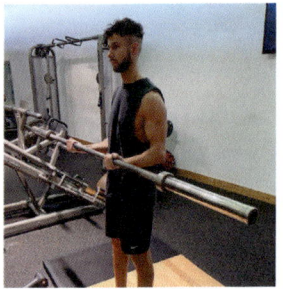

www.abcfit.co.uk

Standing Dumbbell Hammer Curl
Target Areas: Biceps

Stand tall and hold two dumbbells with a neutral grip. Keeping the elbows fixed into your sides, curl the dumbbells up to your chest. Squeeze the biceps to ensure recruitment. Remember to keep it controlled on the way back down.

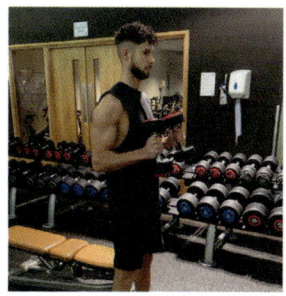

Rope Pressdown
Target Areas: Triceps

Attach a rope to a cable stack. With elbows tucked in by the sides, extend the arm down. Squeeze the triceps at the bottom before returning back up to the start.

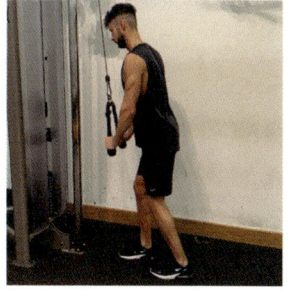

www.abcfit.co.uk

Core

Crunch
Target Areas: Abdominals

Lie supine with your knees slightly bent and feet flat on the ground. Cross your arms over your chest and flex the torso to raise your shoulder blades off the ground. Squeeze the abs at the top of the movement before lowering to the start position. Repeat for reps.

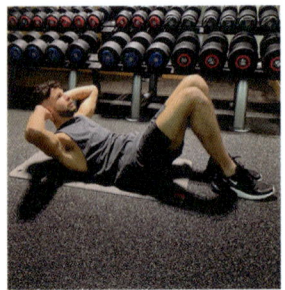

Seated Twist
Target Areas: Obliques

Sit with your knees slightly bent and lean back to a 45 degree angle. Hold a medicine ball and twist side to side. Lift your feet off the ground if you want to make the exercise more challenging.

Coaching Cue - Emphasise the twist. Imagine your chest is following the load all the way around as you twist, this will switch on the target area.

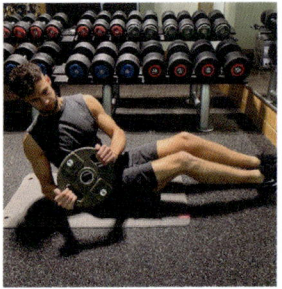

Plank
Target Areas: Abdominals

Hold a bridge position on your elbows and feet. Keep the spine flat and core engaged. Remember to keep breathing for the duration of this movement.

Coaching Cue - Squeeze the glutes to further support the spine.

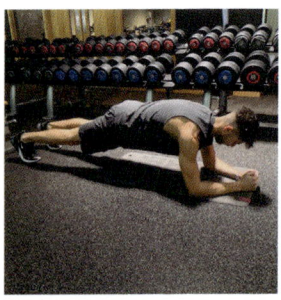

www.abcfit.co.uk

Adapting The Exercises For Home Use

I understand not all of you will have access to a gym and will therfore want to perform the workouts from home with little to no equipment. This is absolutely fine, but I can't stress enough that if you want optimal results a gym with an array of equipment is where it's at. For those wishing to perform the workouts at home, here is each exercise contained within the plan along with a suitable "home" alternative.

Lower Body

Barbell Back Squat - Bodyweight Squat
Dumbbell Romanian Deadlift - Bodyweight Good Morning
Dumbbell Lunge - Bodyweight Lunge
Leg Press - Narrow Stance Bodyweight Squat
Barbell Deadlift - Wide Stance Bodyweight Squat
Back Extension Bench - Prone Skydiver
Seated Leg Curl - Glute Bridge
Leg Extension - Sissy Squat

Upper Body

Seated Dumbbell Press - Inverted Press up
Flat Barbell Press - Press up
Cable Flye - Wide Grip Press Up
Dumbbell Rear Delt Raise - Perform With No Dumbbells
Seated Pulldown - Prone T Raise
One Arm Dumbbell Row - Prone Y Raise
Press Up - Press up
Close Grip Push Up - Close Grip Push Up
Barbell Curl - Towel Curl
Standing Dumbbell Hammer Curl - Towel Curl
Rope Pressdown - Diamond Push Up

Core

Crunch - Crunch
Seated Twist - Seated Twist
Plank - Plank

www.abcfit.co.uk

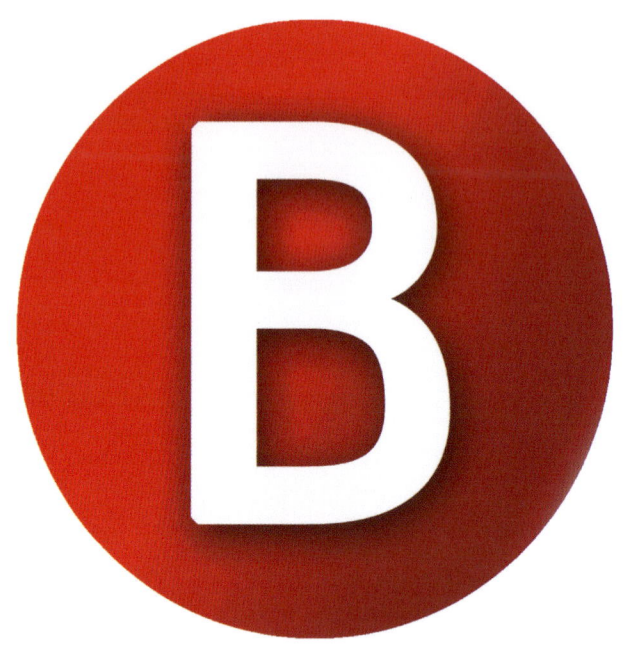

B = NUTRITION

The process of providing or obtaining the food necessary for health and growth

www.abcfit.co.uk

The Seven Principles Of Nutrition

You don't need a meal plan. For long term change and superior results, you need to be educated on the seven principles it takes to build lean muscle mass. The principles below take food to the next level and start to address the macronutrient balance. Using them means you'll take advantage of the hormonal effects of food, nourish your body and never go hungry.

> "How much you eat matters, but the quality of the food we put into our bodies matters more because it drives our gene function, metabolism and health."
> Mark Hyman, MD

Principle #1

Drink 0.033L Of Water Per KG Of Bodyweight Per Day

You're a wet, moving organism made up of around 70% water. The body's ability to digest, transport and absorb nutrients is directly related to your fluid intake. If your tissues become dehydrated they will dry up like desert sand, become sticky and prevent your body from moving in an optimal range. With dehydration comes a decrease in work capacity by up to 30%. Prevent this by consuming 0.033L of water per KG of bodyweight per day.

For a 75kg individual this would be:

0.033L x 75 = 2.4L per day

Consider spiking your drinking water with electrolytes to expedite absorption.

Principle #2

Eat Four Medium Meals/Snacks A Day

The evidence surrounding eating little and often is somewhat sketchy, but for whatever reason it seems to work for most people. Eating often is also important for sustained energy levels as it helps keep blood sugar levels stable, as well as potentially helping to preserve and build lean muscle mass.

www.abcfit.co.uk

Principle #3

Remove Sugar/Processed Foods From The Diet
A good question to ask yourself before you put something in your mouth is "would this have existed 5000 years ago?" If the answer is no, you probably shouldn't eat it (excluding the supplements that we'll get onto later). Processed foods often contain high amounts of trans-fats, salt, sugar and preservatives. None of which are going to be a major contributor to your muscle gain goals. High sugar foods give a steep rise in blood sugar levels and a surge of insulin, followed by an energy crash. Constant crashes in blood sugar and excess insulin will lead chronically raised levels of the stress hormone cortisol and insulin resistance. For building lean body mass we need to use nutrition to our advantage and become sensitive to insulin. The diagram below shows two possible scenarios. If 10-30g of carbohydrates is optimal for blood sugar levels, on the left we can see what happens when a high sugar diet is consumed. Blood sugar levels are sent on a roller coaster ride. The right hand side shows an ideal scenario - blood sugar levels are much more controlled and glucagon is stimulated when blood sugar is at a low point. By following the seven principles laid out in this manual you will achieve this.

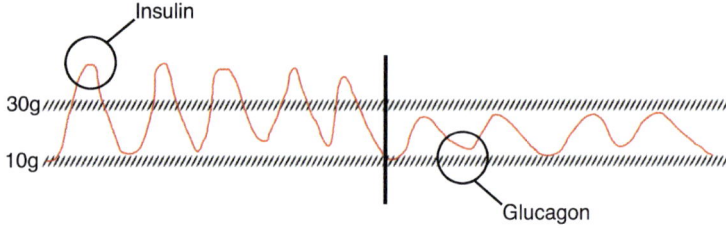

What Is Insulin?
Insulin is a hormone made by the pancreas and is often described as the key that unlocks a cell to allow glucose (blood sugar) to enter. In the diagram above, insulin is being released to clear up all of the excess blood sugar. When it's cleared up it usually gets stored away in adipocytes/fat cells. Controlling carbohydrates and choosing the correct types will help us develop insulin sensitivity. This means the body won't have to produce as much insulin for it to have an efficient effect.

What Is Glucagon?
Glucagon is stimulated by protein. It works in an opposite way to insulin, in the respect that it can elevate the levels of glucose in the blood for sustained energy levels and help the body to burn fat.

www.abcfit.co.uk

Principle #4

Consume A Hand Sized Portion Of Greens At Every Meal

Vegetables and leafy greens should be consumed in abundance throughout the day. Don't worry about breakfast, but with every other meal at least half of your plate should be covered with greens. They're high in fibre, low in calories and are an important source of many nutrients, including potassium, folic acid, vitamin A and vitamin C.

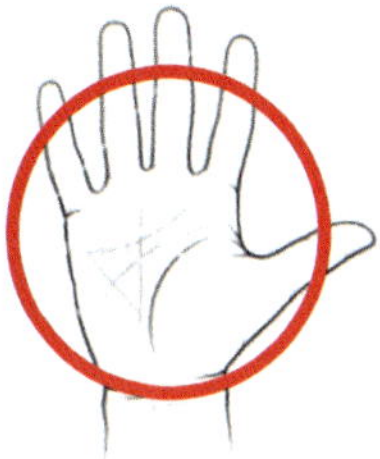

Greens have their highest nutrient content right after they're picked. So always opt for fresh, organic produce where you can. When it comes to cooking your greens, you can steam, boil or wilt. Whichever mehod you choose be careful not to overcook them. Overcooked greens will be robbed of many nutrients.

Ensure your diet regularly contains the following:

Broccoli
Spinach
Kale
Garden peas
Asparagus
Cabbage
Lettuce
Collards
Green beans

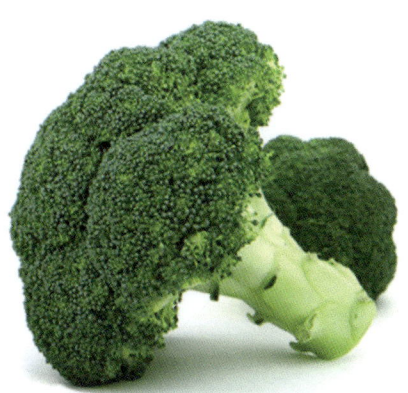

www.abcfit.co.uk

Principle #5

Consume 1-2 Palm Size Portions Of Protein Per Meal

Protein plays a vital role in the body, especially when it comes to burning fat and maintaining lean body mass. Proteins are complex substances, that are broken down into amino acids and rearranged into new proteins that your body needs. Protein is quite hard for the body to digest, meaning you'll feel fuller for longer. It also stimulates glucagon, a hormone that raises the levels of glucose in the bloodstream and helps you burn fat for fuel.

A palm sized portion of protein will roughly contain 20-30g of protein. Based on four meals per day, a female should consume one palm sized portion of protein with each meal, whereas a male should aim for two.

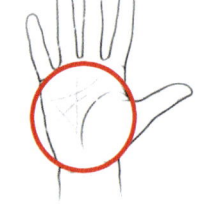

Choose your protein sources from the following list:

Chicken
Eggs
Turkey
Salmon
Tuna
Swordfish
Mackerel
Sea bass
Sardines
Trout
Prawns
Crab
Lobster
Cod
Beef
Venison
Buffalo
Ostrich
Zebra
Whey protein shake

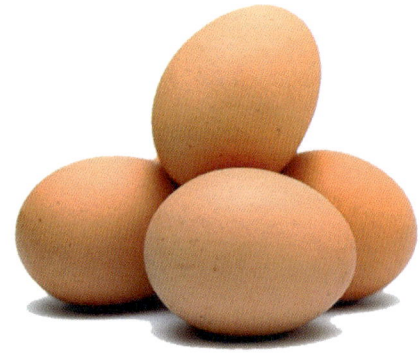

www.abcfit.co.uk

Principle #6

Eat Carbohydrates At Every Meal

Carbohydrates are your body's most important source of energy. We need energy for movement, growth and repair. You've already learned that simple sugars are bad news for blood sugar level control, so you should be looking to mainly consume complex carbohydrates.

Aim to consume a fist sized portion of carbs with each of your meals. If you're an individual that struggles to gain weight, consider having two fist sized portions with each of your meals.

Sweet potato
Brown bread
White bread
Wraps
Cereal
Granola
Yam
Quinoa
Brown rice
Brown pasta
White potato
Blueberries
Strawberries
Raspberries
Apples
Bananas
Pears

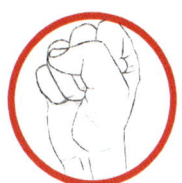

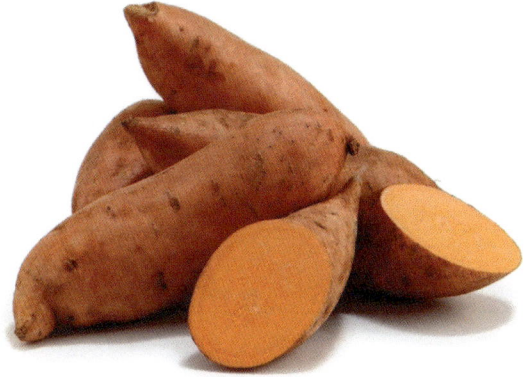

www.abcfit.co.uk

Principle #7

Consume A Thumb Sized Portion Of Fat With Every Meal

Don't fear fat! Fats are needed in the body to help absorb various nutrients, nourish the nervous system, maintain cell structures and regulate hormone levels. Fats are also fairly hard for the body to break down meaning they can keep you feeling fuller for longer. Trans-fats should be avoided.

Aim for a thumb sized portion of fat with every meal. This equates to around 10-15g of fat. Breaking this down further it could be something like a tablespoon of coconut oil to cook with, a tablespoon of olive oil as a dressing on your greens or a small portion of nuts.

Ensure your healthy fat sources include the following:

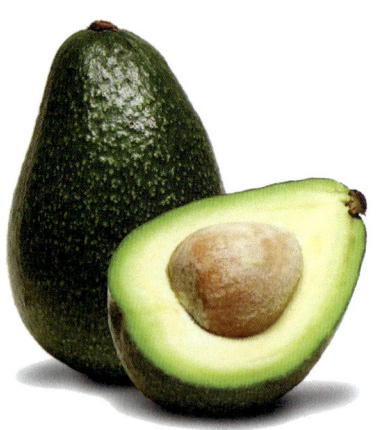

Coconut oil
Avocados
Plain nuts
Cheese
Seeds
Olive oil
Hazelnut oil
Avocado oil
Flax oil

If you can hand on heart say you're abiding by the seven principles above and still not getting anywhere, either you're not training hard enough, or you're not consuming enough calories. You may need to re-evaluate that you are properly abiding by the portion size guidelines of the principles.

www.abcfit.co.uk

Supplements

Once the seven principles of nutrition are understood and put into practice, you then have the option to incorporate supplements. Remember a supplement is only as good as your nutrition, but with that said the correct supplement protocol can produce exceedingly good quality sessions, assist with building muscle and promote a rapid recovery. The muscle gain supplement market is a minefield of false advertising and fads. All of the supplements mentioned below are backed by science and produce results.

Creatine
How Much:
5g per day
Function:

Start off with taking 5g of creatine either before or after your workout. Creatine is an organic compound found in red meat and is one of the most researched supplements around. It's the number one supplement for improving performance in the gym. It's primary role is to increase the stores in the muscle cells meaning the additional stores and be used to produce more ATP which is the key energy source for heavy lifting and high-intensity exercise.

Omega 3s
How Much:
2-4g a day
Function:

Omega 3s contain the fatty acids EPA and DHA. Split your daily dose into two and take half with breakfast and half with your evening meal. They deliver some amazing health benefits such as heart health, joint health, brain function, bone health, regulation of your cholesterol triglyceride levels, helping to reduce post-exercise inflammation, lowering of the stress hormone cortisol, improving insulin sensitivity, speeding up metabolism, improving digestion and promoting healthy skin and hair.

Whey Protein
How Much:
20-30g
Function:

If you're struggling to acheive your goal of 1-2 palm sized portions of protein with each meal, try adding in whey protein powder as a supplement. It's great way to deliver some amino acids to your repairing muscles and conveniently top-up your protein intake levels.

www.abcfit.co.uk

A Day In The Life

Now you have a better understanding of the seven princinples of nutrition and supplements for a better body, here's how they come together. This is what a typical day might look like for an individual training in the evening after school or college.

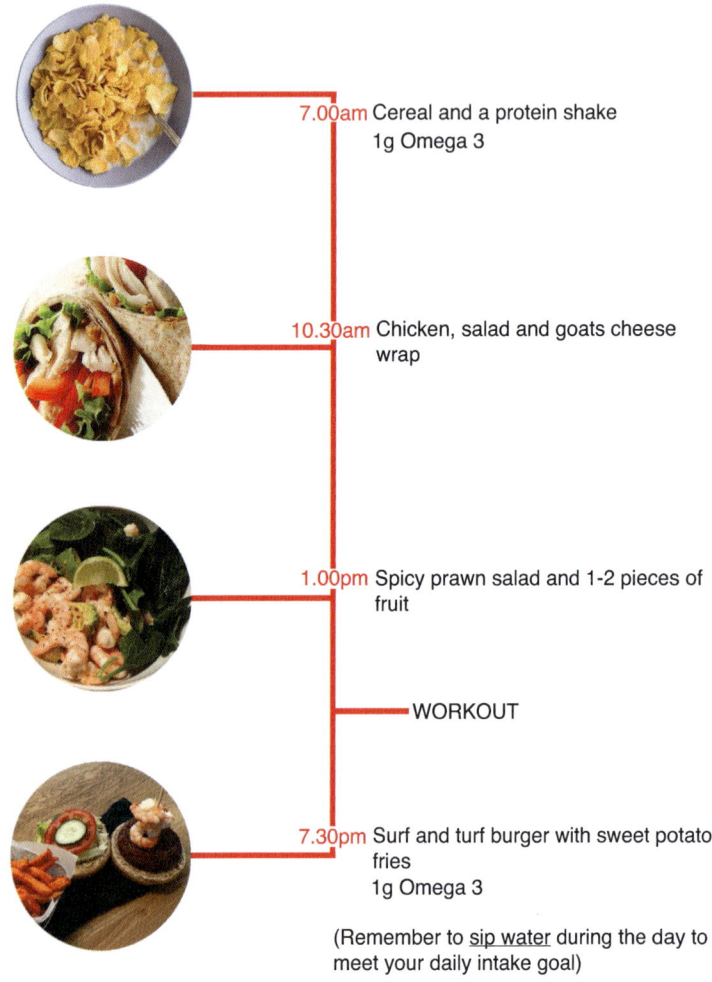

7.00am Cereal and a protein shake
        1g Omega 3

10.30am Chicken, salad and goats cheese wrap

1.00pm Spicy prawn salad and 1-2 pieces of fruit

WORKOUT

7.30pm Surf and turf burger with sweet potato fries
        1g Omega 3

(Remember to sip water during the day to meet your daily intake goal)

www.abcfit.co.uk

The 80/20 Rule

No one is perfect! Not even me.

And I'm not expecting you to be either. Telling you to follow the principles presented in this manual to the letter, with no exceptions is outdated advice.

If you follow the principles previously mentioned 80% of the time, you'll see some decent results. The extra 20% gives you some flexibility to eat out on weekends or go to a party etc. To make this work and not affect your progress, you just need to plan ahead. For example, eat less during the day if you know you'll be eating/drinking a lot more in the evening. This way you can still keep on track with your muscle building goals and not end up binge eating so much you gain too much fat!

Typical Weekday Eating

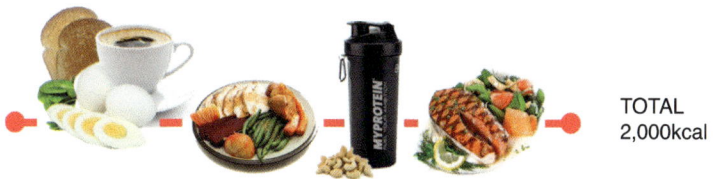

TOTAL
2,000kcal

Smart Weekend Eating

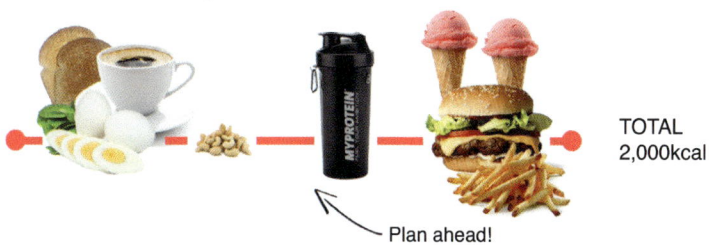

TOTAL
2,000kcal

Plan ahead!

It's really that simple, but you'd be surprised how many people forget to do it. The infographic gives you a perfect example of how this works.

www.abcfit.co.uk

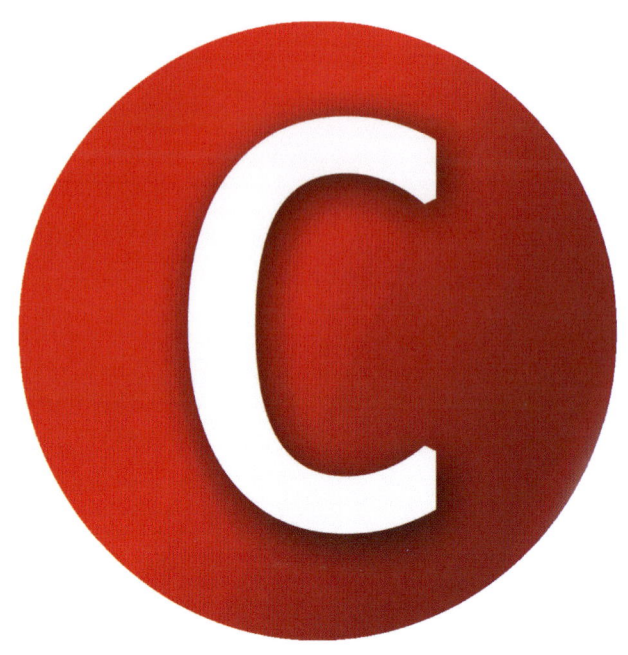

C = RECOVERY

A return to a normal state of health, mind or strength

Sleep Fundamentals

A good night's sleep of 8-9 hours is paramount for optimal recovery, not only from exercise, but from everyday life as well. Accumulating evidence from epidemiological studies and well-controlled lab studies indicate lack of sleep may increase weight gain and impair muscle growth. Since your goals include increasing lean muscle mass, you need to be taking sleep seriously. Lack of sleep also results in metabolic and endocrine alterations such as decreased insulin sensitivity, raised levels of the stress hormone cortisol during the evening, increased levels of ghrelin (a hunger hormone), decreased levels of leptin (a satiety hormone) and lowered release of human Growth Hormone (GH).

Turning your bedroom into a batcave, by keeping it cool, dark and free of all electronic distractions such as phones, TV's and radios etc. will really improve your sleep quality. Having a curfue of say 10.00pm or 10.30pm is also wise as a good night's sleep is essentially a good habit and this curfue will reinforce it. Once you're in bed take a moment to be thankful for everyone and everything you have in your life. It's much easier to fall asleep being at peace. A final word of advice is to avoid stimulants in the evenings. Nothing upsets your natural sleep cycle like a big dose of caffeine in the evening. Eliminate all teas, coffees and other stimulant/high caffeinated drinks after 3pm.

The Sleep/Wake Cycle

Many of our hormones are produced in tune with the cycle of the sun. Stress hormones (such as cortisol) and growth/repair hormones (such as GH) will work in opposition to each other. For the majority, a typical day involves highly elevated stress levels. You might be late for school, you forgot to eat breakfast, your teacher wanted that report finished last week and your mum wants you to do your homework! (Trust me when I say I've been there too). All of this can result in increased levels of stress hormones during the day, resulting in decreased levels of growth/repair hormones. This will have a huge impact on your recovery rate. Notice how on the diagram below stress hormone (black line) levels stay elevated for a long duration of time, not leaving much time for the growth/repair hormones (white line) to do their thing. Follow the tips above and you'll lower stress hormones, and increase the growth/repair hormones.

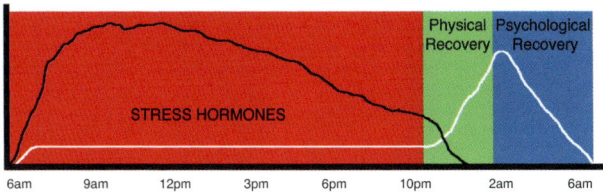

www.abcfit.co.uk

Active Recovery

With the correct exercise and nutritional protocol in place, there's one last thing you need to get in check to see maximal results. Your ability to recover is largely dependant on your nutritional status and hours of sleep you've had. So at the very least you should be abiding by the seven principles of nutrition 80% of the time and getting 8-9 hours of sleep per night.

Types Of Recovery

Tissue Repair - Microscopic tissue damage from exercise is repaired. Explaining how this process happens is beyond the scope of this manual, but you should know that it is through this process the muscle tissues grow back bigger and stronger (hypertrophy).

Function Restoration - Joints and tissues return to a state of optimal function. Healthy tissues should slide and glide over each other (known as sliding surface function). This keeps the body moving in an optimal range.

Muscle Recovery - Muscles return to normal length and state.

Psychological Recovery - Head is strong, focused and motivation to train remains on a high.

CNS Recovery - Central Nervous System makes a full recovery. Heavy, intense weight training sessions can be quite fatiguing for the CNS.

In order to maximise recovery I've put together The Active Recovery Session. It's a short 10 minute session that should be performed one or two times per week. Your returns on investment from that 10 minutes will be huge. Perform session whenever you can - post-workout, in the garden, at school, at home in the evening in front of the TV etc. The tasks are designed to speed up all of the main types of recovery, not only from exercise, but from everyday life as well. The session will address all of the common areas of the body that tend to get glued up. Before we look at the session, lets take a look at the guidelines you need to understand and follow:

- Practice good positions (keep your spine tall and core lightly braced).
- Spend 30-45 seconds on each.
- Breathe deep and relax.

www.abcfit.co.uk

Hip Flexor Stretch

This drill captures the tissues of the anterior hip and quads. Sitting for extended periods will result in a tight hip flexor complex that will rock the pelvis forward, moving it into an anterior tilt. This changes our posture and places a great deal of pressure on the lumbar spine. Start in a kneeling position, and push your hips into it. Hold for 30 seconds per side.

Progressions
- Elevate the back foot

Regressions
- Less push forward into it

Hamstring Stretch

The hamstrings are responsible for two very important jobs - knee flexion and hip extension. Tightness in the hamstrings, if not taken care of, can cause knee pain and lower back pain. Begin with feet wide apart and reach forward aiming to touch your toes. Breathe deep and relax into it. Hold for 30 seconds.

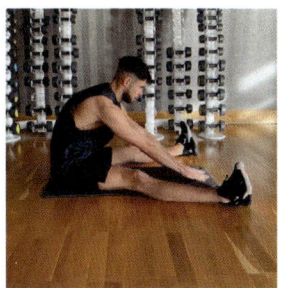

Progressions
- Wider feet
- Further reach

Regressions
- Closer feet
- Less of a reach

www.abcfit.co.uk

T-Spine Foam Roll

The thoracic spine is a pretty common area to get stiff. If you spend your day bolted to a chair at school etc. your spine slowly rounds forward into a kyphotic C shape. This drill will create a large global extension through the T-spine and as a result will improve posture, thoracic mobility and shoulder positioning. To begin, place the roller at the base of the ribcage. With your feet and bum firmly on the ground support your head and relax back into it. Slowly roll up and down. Spend 60-90 seconds on this drill.

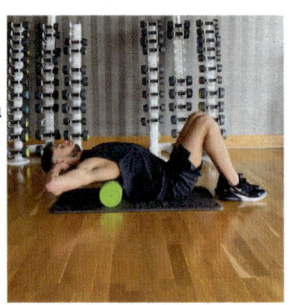

Progressions
- Reach your arms above your head

Regressions
- No rolling up and down. Just hold the position

Chest Stretch

Tightness across the chest and anterior shoulder complex will drag the scapula forward to create poor posture and pain. Once again this area tends to get pretty glued up from extended periods of sitting. Kneel down, place your hands on your bum and try to draw the elbows together until you feel the stretch across the chest. Hold for 30 seconds.

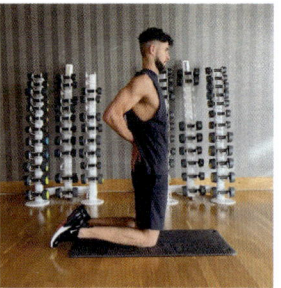

Progressions
- Draw elbows closer

Regressions
- Don't draw elbows as close together

www.abcfit.co.uk

FAQs

I can't train on the days suggested on the workout diary, does it matter?
No. In an ideal world you would, as the sessions have been placed to allow enough recovery time between sessions. They also give you the weekends off, but if you can't just do what you can. As long as you get all of your sessions in for that week.

What time of the day should I train?
Don't overthink this, train whenever you can/feel best. I would however, strongly urge you don't exercise first thing in the morning on an empty stomach. Contrary to popular belief, training in a fasted state won't guarantee you'll burn more fat. It will mean you'll have a rubbish workout and be more likley to tap into lean body mass for fuel.

Why am I finding the workouts too easy?
The sets, reps, times, rests and tempos have all been programmed to support the goals of the training phase you're in. If you're finding the sessions too easy, make sure you're lifting a heavy enough weight that allows you to complete the desired number of reps, but no more, and be super strict with the tempos and rest periods between sets.

I noticed you recommend a warm-up before the workouts, but what about a cool-down after?
Your cool-down for these programs is to hit the shower and then eat some food. The active recovery drills outlined in section C will speed up recovery and take care of keeping your tissues flexible and healthy. This is even more reason to give the recovery section as much attention as the exercise and nutrition.

What makes it easier to stick to a diet or certain way of eating in the long run?
There's two key things that will make any diet plan stick. Here they are in order of importance.

1) Enjoyment - If you enjoy the foods you're eating, you'll be more likely to stick to it. If you hate them it's only a matter of time before you'll give it all up.

2) Results - If you notice results, you'll enjoy it more!

www.abcfit.co.uk

Help, I'm really struggling! Why can't I seem to stick to this?
Following an ebook like this, may not be for everyone. You may need some closer guidance, more accountability and a little push along the way. If this sounds like you, the online coaching packages with ABC fit would be perfect for your needs. Head to www.abcfit.co.uk and send me an enquiry.

What shoes are best to workout in?
In all honesty, something simple with a flat sole is best. Examples include Converse and Vans. If you want something a little more "flash" I really like the Nike Metcons.

What if I miss a workout?
That's ok, don't beat yourself up over it. Just get back on it at the next nearest available opportunity.

Can I get abs on this plan?
Yes! Absolutely. If you want abs you need to create an energy deficit to burn off excess fat revealing the abs hidden underneath. Follow the nutritional principles laid out in the manual, but look at reducing portion sizes of meals to help create this energy deficit.

I'm really struggling with the food side of things. Any tips?
Planning and prep is everything! Make meals and pack lunches the evening before the following day etc. Get your parents and your friends on board with your goals and get them to support you.

Man down! I've sustained an injury. Should I carry on training?
Firstly, listen to your body. Leave your ego behind and don't push through pain. If it's really hurting take a week off from your training, but really focus on your nutrition and the active recovery drills presented in the guide.

Is it good to have achy muscles the day following a workout?
I know it feels good, it feels like you've actually had a great workout, but don't be upset if you don't. Despite being somewhat indicative of how much muscle damage you did, it's not the be all and end all of a good session.

I've finished the programme, what now?
You can start it over. Start again with the goal setting activity and work through phases one, two and three like before. As a means of progression, look to lift more than your first cycle. Or check out the Lean Body Academy with ABC fit. It's a monthly subscription service that gives you access to heaps of useful content and a new, workout plan every month: https://abcfit.co.uk/lean-body-academy/

Basic Anatomy

If you didn't pay attention in biology class, no worries! You can catch up now. It's important to understand which muscle groups each exercise is targeting, so you can refer to this chart if you need to.

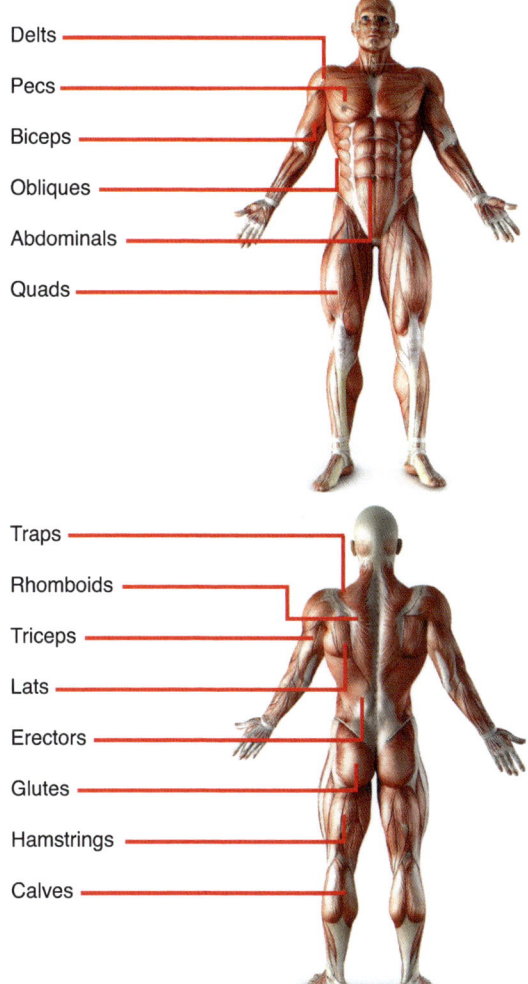

- Delts
- Pecs
- Biceps
- Obliques
- Abdominals
- Quads

- Traps
- Rhomboids
- Triceps
- Lats
- Erectors
- Glutes
- Hamstrings
- Calves

www.abcfit.co.uk

Enjoyed The Programme?

Share your experiences and results with us on...

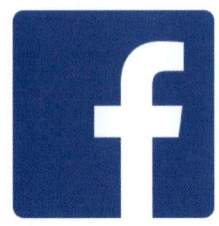

www.facebook.com/abcfit3

@abcfit3

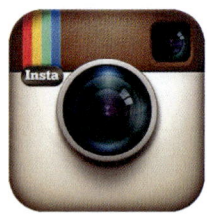

@abcfit3

#ABCFIT #8WEEKTMP

www.abcfit.co.uk

Maximise your results with...

ONLINE COACHING

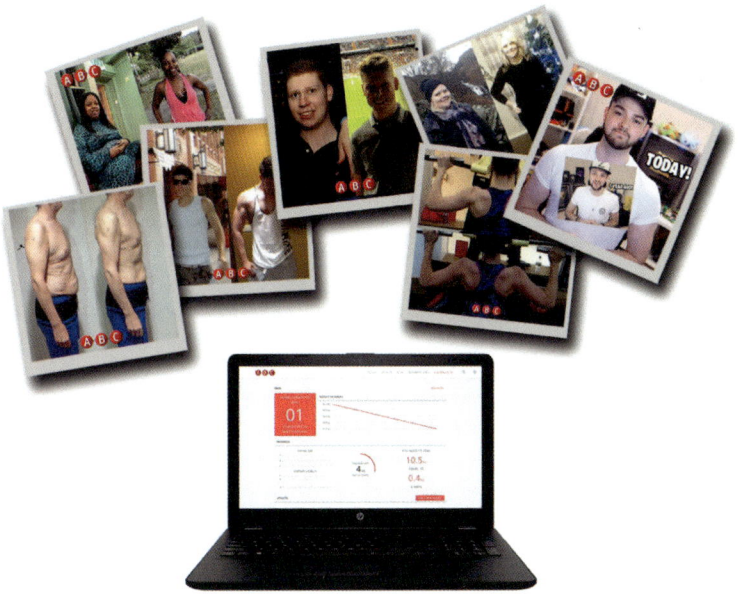

Tailored diet plans based on your goal and preferences. We can be specific to your likes and dislikes also go into detail based on your allergies, time for cooking, money for grocery shopping and more.

Tailored programme based on your goals and specific requirements.

You get 1-to-1 coaching from me including video chat and regular personal updates.

You will get your own online page, where you have to do weekly check-ins. My goal is to help you reach yours! Based on your progression I will change your diet and training every 4 weeks.

Apply now at
www.abcfit.co.uk

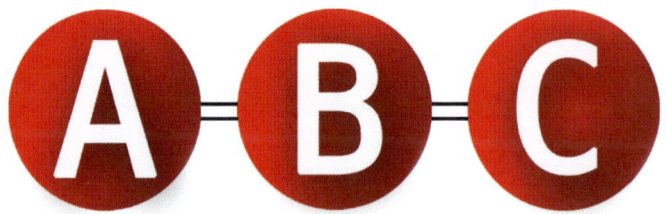

www.abcfit.co.uk

ABC fit was created by Aaron Breckell. Aaron's passion for health and fitness was first ignited at the age of 18, when he entered the gym at 6ft and 54kg. Exercise, nutrition and recovery not only changed his body, his entire life changed for the better too. Since it all started he has modelled for various supplement and underwear companies and was successfully shortlisted down to the final six in the Maximuscle Body of the Year contest 2010. With over five years fitness industry experience, Aaron has successfully worked with a wide array of clientele including CEO's, doctors, competitive athletes and YouTube superstars. This is his way of easily sharing with you the information it takes to achieve the fitness success you truly deserve.

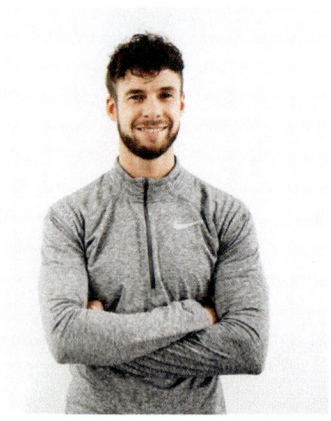